Chapter 14: Final Thoughts & Next Steps

CHAPTER 1: WHY I WANT TO SHARE WITH YOU MY EXPERIENCE RAISING A CHILD WITH ADD/ADHD

Thank you, for taking the time to read my story and hear what I have to say about one of the most vulnerable times in my life.

As a parent, I've learned how my stubbornness and lack of education surrounding ADD/ADHD, hurt my relationship with my son Keagan.

For as long as I can remember, I was in the dark about the therapy available to properly support him. Instead, what I thought was "helping" my son, actually aided in his struggles.

My hopes in sharing this chapter of my life with you by writing this book, not only helps you avoid some of the pitfalls I jumped into (head first), but also gain some comfort in knowing you are adding tools to your mom (or dad) toolbox.

Further, this is not to force my views on you, but simply to share with you a breakthrough we finally had after nearly 23 years of butting heads, spinning in a lack of confidence and driving a wedge in between my son and me...

ADD/ADHD has been called a condition, a disease, a mental illness, an excuse, a myth, a distraction . . . and, on and on.

This book is not to label ADD/ADHD in ANY fashion.

It is simply to share my journey.

My shortcomings. My triumphs. My lessons...

Because, in this life, we often walk through it thinking we're alone, or that we're going to be judged, or that we're the only ones dealt this particular deck of cards.

We battle questions. We battle opinions and advice. We listen to and question medical professionals. We run down paths, full-speed looking for the best answers.

Chasing Monday, praying for Friday, and wondering all along . . . am I doing this the right way?

Like I've said again and again. If and when, there is a book on how to be the "perfect" parent, sign me up... but thankfully that is never going to happen or exist, so we can all relax, we're all in a safe space here.

So again, my deepest wish is not only that this book reminds you that you are NOT alone, but also that it reminds you, that you are doing the best you can, and that it is truly the only thing a child (or loved one) needs from you.

… And the same goes for you.

So, before we go any further, I'm going to take you back to those earlier days of our family life.

For the record, just to be clear, I am NOT a medical professional and I hold no licenses in medicine. I am a mom, a wife, a daughter, a sister, a cousin, an aunt, and a friend that goes through life based on logic, research and an ever-burning desire to learn and grow. This is my story, not a medical directive.

Now that we got that out of the way, let's take it back a few decades. ;)

CHAPTER 2: THOSE CURIOUS ABOUT ALTERNATE METHODS FOR ADD/ADHD ROADBLOCKS (AND HOW TO OVERCOME THEM)

I don't think of myself as an expert. But, I guess when you say or hear "expert" we often think of someone with a Ph.D. behind his or her name.

When I think of "expert", I think of someone who has experienced, lived through or with the topic that's being discussed. Someone who is able to share advice on, and/or information. A topic they've become wise in.

What better way to know about this particular topic than to have been living with those that suffer from ADD or feeling that, I myself, might suffer from ADD as well?

I wasn't really aware of what ADD or ADHD was or what it stood for until I met my ex-husband, Sean.

He had ADHD (Attention Deficit Hyperactivity Disorder), and now looking back it's funny to think that what I really liked about him, was his endless energy, his spontaneity and lack of focus, he was like an amusement park.

Crazy, right?

We rebelled quite a bit in our younger years and as immature as we were, a lot of his tendencies were due to his "condition"... I understand that it was partially due to age, but little did I know that ADHD was the reason for most of the traits he had.

The enormous and wild ideas, some that were so left field that I couldn't comprehend where they were coming from, not to mention the always-on-the-go demeanor... it was attractive. I liked it.

These traits kept me running. But, in time, these were the exact same traits that destroyed our relationship and unfortunately, he eventually could not be settled without substance.

If you're reading this book, my guess is, you know what the "symptoms" or "signs" of ADHD are, but what may be hidden a bit beyond the surface is, these traits can cause havoc on one's life, and those around them.

It took me years, to understand all of this, I just kept asking myself, how could someone I love so much... drive me this crazy?

This "condition" is something that causes people to be extremely unfocused, and struggle with all sorts of teachings, from classroom environments to basic life lessons.

Many have anxiety, develop depression, turn to substance abuse and can't seem to relax. Many can't even tolerate someone else with ADHD.

They're "scattered" as people would call them, very outspoken, and many don't think before they act, rarely have a filter, taking things a little too far.

These are traits that often calm down in later years for many, but this was my first interaction and learning of ADD/ADHD.

We were very young when we started having children. I was 20 and Sean was 19 and I had only heard of the struggles that Sean had gone through as a child.

Our kids are now 24 and 23 but imagine having twins at such a young age. We had a boy and a girl, who was born at Christmas time in 1994 and then a year later, in January of 1996, we had another daughter. We were barely getting by and at the best of times, just simply trying to keep it all together, so with being new parents times 3 in a matter of 13 months, we had a lot going on.

They say don't compare your children, but when you have twins, it's really hard not too and it didn't take us long to learn that one had ADHD, the other didn't.

We could tell that our son had ADHD at a very young age, and that's where I started educating myself on what our options were.

I knew that Sean hated being on Ritalin, how it made him feel, and disliking who he was when on it. He wasn't himself; he referred to it like a drugged "version" of himself.

I knew of his strained relationships of all sorts, his troubles in school, the conflict with his parents and then, of course, use of the drug Ritalin.

In the 90's the only alternative I knew of seemed to be diet and Ritalin, and I knew I did not want to put Keagan on drugs.

I also had a history with drugs and I learned that Ritalin was something that some searched out as a method of abuse and addiction.

Sean and I both had addictive personalities. Although a painful truth, we knew it was our truth. Even more so, we knew it was not a choice we wanted for our kids. Sean would describe himself as feeling like a zombie when on Ritalin, and we just didn't want Keagan, to experience that feeling.

When I first started doing my research on what else I could do to help Keagan instead of putting him on prescription drugs, I found therapy, but it wasn't until about school age when we began looking into what we could do to help him socialize, get along with others and focus confidently at school.

We couldn't afford much but I knew there was counseling that needed to be done. We also knew there was additional schooling that would be required to help him catch up before and after school and with tutors.

We managed to get him a private tutor and in grade 1 we had to make the decision to have Keagan held back a year. As much as we could, we let him make the decision so that he could be involved.

But - having a twin sister . . . in the same grade. Well, let's just say, it was not easy.

Thankfully the school kept them in a 1- 2 split class, but there were still conflicts, comparisons and insecurity issues to combat and defuse.

Our son was very hyperactive and he couldn't focus. Not only at school, but even with simple requests at home.

After pulling out every stop we could think of, we finally stopped and asked ourselves "Okay, now what?"

... Again, I turned to diet and I talked to some of my family members that had experience with ADD and Ritalin at the same time, and again and again, it turned to diet, so I kept Keagan off of as much sugar as I possibly could.

We kept it consistent for all three, which wasn't a bad thing. They'd all still get their favorite cereal at Christmas and on Birthdays and of course candy at Halloween, but we really tried to keep it away as it didn't help Keagan at all.

Our kids weren't sent to school with all of the other treats that a lot of the other kids were, but I'm sure they would sneak or trade. At one point I was thanked by some of their teachers that I didn't send them with sugary treats.

I think that it was a much bigger issue than so many of us knew.

Despite the huge sugar limitations, he still struggled extensively. At times, I kept asking myself, do I have to put him on prescriptions? I KNEW I did not want to, but in all honesty, it was still a question I struggled with myself. Bad.

I often felt like I was stuck in between a rock and a hard place, and if I put him on Ritalin, the drug his dad says zombie-fys him, I will take away his personality, the determination and natural sense of my son.

On the contrary, I sat there trying to help him sort through his frustrations, his lack of focus and added challenges when "compared" to society's idealistic behaviors at each respective age.

With report cards, we got a lot of "needs to improve", "not focused in class" and "not paying attention" etc... and that was a really difficult struggle for us. Was it all ADD or was he just challenged academically? I was terrible in school and struggled extensively, where Sean did quite well and also graduated, I-DID-NOT.

We kept him really active in sports, but again, he struggled with his social skills.

He frequently found ways to get in trouble and be a troublemaker and even though he wasn't a bad kid or mean by any stretch, he followed the pack. He was much more easily influenced than his twin sister.

I'm sure it didn't help that Sean and I were separated even before the kids started school. They were 3 and 4, and that added a lot to the equation. However, I would definitely say the social struggles were the hardest for sure.

No one wants to see their child struggle that way, and that is one of the biggest struggles for kids let alone those with these added challenges.

Other kids don't understand ADD and people don't relate to ADD unless it affects them. Those with ADD/ADHD can be so hyper and have a really hard time focusing. Social awkwardness is common and results in our little ones questioning themselves, adding to the distractions they face.

Reading is a struggle. I knew of the struggles of re-read things over and over again, your mind is racing and going in a million different directions. You just can't focus.

Not only did he struggle throughout school, despite being incredibly intelligent, any tasks that took extreme focus . . . well, let's just say . . . most times he found himself sitting in the front of the classroom and bringing home extra homework. (Or shall I say, school work he didn't finish.)

With sports, he was all over the place, and again, had a hard time focusing, but hockey and soccer suited him best. Other sports not-so-much. Some sports suit some children with ADD/ADHD and others do not, and as we all know, even at the best of times.

Then there was the bullying and a general sense of being less than . . . with being held-back, an often "troublemaker" and socially awkward . . . it was a daily focus point of mine to help him manage, but, we know, how much easier said than done that is.

Don't we all wish that we had the ability to protect our children 24/7? I remember thinking over and over again how I wished I could have kept my kids in a bubble, but I knew how sheltered and unrealistic that is... I just couldn't believe how people can be so cruel. Still can't.

CHAPTER 3: A CRITICAL AH-HA MOMENT

I find that all those experiences and that past history with all of the struggles I went through, changed me as a parent.

But, trust me, Keagan and I butted heads a lot.

We had a lot of issues as just a mother/son relationship because I didn't have the patience that I needed to with his certain tendencies.

It didn't help that I was ALWAYS working when the kids were young and they needed more attention, but I find now, more than ever, I can relate more and understand more.

It also opened my eyes up to actually becoming more educated and stop being so ignorant to alternative methods, something that Keagan had been trying to talk to me about for years!

Within this last year, in a casual conversation with a friend, it was mentioned about this cream she used for her extreme back pain. As we dug into the conversation more, she mentioned that it had CBD in it, and as soon as she said it, the conversation I had with Keagan came to mind.

He mentioned how CBD oil was helping him with anxiety, his ADD, pain relief, sleep, and a general sense of well being. Keagan had mentioned repeatedly how it was helping HIM.

But, of course, as soon as she said CBD... I thought, drugs, the same thing I thought when Keagan said it. I thought about our addictive personalities. I thought about everything I had lost and given up on in my life because of drugs.

Then, the conversation with my girlfriend progressed. She told me how in 2016 before her back surgery the CBD cream helped her more than heavy prescription painkillers. Then she went on to say that every nerve ending in our body naturally has a receptor for CBD (the cannabinoid derived from the hemp plant).

Before she could get the words out of my mouth, it was like fireworks were happening for me.

My mind was racing and I started researching it... more and more and more.

Soon, I learned why CBD was helping SO MANY things for SO MANY people. Once I learned it was naturally something our bodies need and use to process every nerve signal . . . all I could think was . . .

I suck.

I should've listened to Keagan a long time ago.

A LONG TIME AGO...

CHAPTER 4: FIRST MAJOR BREAKTHROUGH WITH HOW I LEARNED TO UNDERSTAND MY SON & HIS USE OF CBD

Unfortunately, I still wasn't convinced entirely despite hearing or finding nothing but good things within my research. I could not get the concept out of my head that it was not a drug.

Then, soon enough, I could not ignore it anymore. Canada was changing their laws on it. My son was having magnificent benefits because of it (more on that soon), and then . . . a number of my friends began using it and selling it.

I guess that was the straw that caused the "major breakthrough". If so many others are ok with it, why can't I be?

And, you know, I know, you know . . . that sometimes . . . this is what it takes before we change our minds about things, but I'm going to be brutally honest with you and say that this initially piqued my interest due to a business opportunity...

Again, I suck. So...

I went back to research.

I remember having to do a ton of research about the products themselves and the differences between the Hemp and the Marijuana plants.

Along the way, I found many people who knew what they were

talking about. I also found a lot of the opposite.

There were some that just wanted to make a dollar and not actually learn about what they were selling, and there were others that had no idea that CBD could be beneficial without THC, or, that there were different plants that it was derived from.

The money intrigued me at first, but I would never get involved with a product like this without knowing how I could help people and what this product could do for those interested. I needed to know the guts of it all.

Among so many other misconceptions, misleading info and noise, I continued my pursuit to truly understand the research. The success stories, the cancer survivors, the pain-free benefits people were experiencing, the sense of calm and presence I had FINALLY seen in my son.

Finally, I said enough is enough.

I don't need paper, a commercial or a salesperson to tell me the details.

I needed to simply look at my son.

And, from that moment forward, what others thought, said, understood or judged me for, meant nothing.

Seeing my son feel like he loved his own skin . . . that was all I needed. I'm not saying that it was a miracle solution to everything, but it was a great start.

CHAPTER 5: WHAT DID I LEARN?

Before, we go any further . . . heads up, here comes a little techno-babble . . . but after we get through the technical stuff, we will go back to English ;)

The human body has what is called an endocannabinoid system inside our brains and nervous systems. According to Wikipedia, "The endocannabinoid system (ECS) is a biological system composed of endocannabinoids, which are endogenous lipid-based retrograde neurotransmitters that bind to cannabinoid receptors, and cannabinoid receptor proteins that are expressed throughout the mammalian central nervous system (including the brain) and peripheral nervous system."

The endocannabinoid system is involved in regulating a variety of physiological and cognitive processes including fertility, pregnancy during pre- and postnatal development, appetite, pain-sensation, mood, and memory, and in mediating the pharmacological effects of cannabis."

That's quite a mouthful of technical and medical jargon, isn't it?

Here's what it means in plain English: your body and central nervous system are actually DESIGNED to work with cannabinoids.

Because of that, hemp is a true wonder of nature. No, we probably don't need the THC found in marijuana (although it MAY have some health benefits), but we do need the benefits of the many cannabinoids found in hemp, especially CBD!

While I must refrain from making any medical claims for CBD oil, there is a large body of medical and scientific research outlining the many benefits of this natural product.

Others are reporting relief and help for a wide variety of health issues.

According to Cannabis research firm Brightfield Group, the CBD market will be a $5.7 billion market by next year, and a $22 billion market by 2022.

What does that mean?

It means we are finally catching on.

It means we are remembering how many benefits we used to enjoy by using the plant correctly.

We have sports teams, the news, doctors, all talking about CBD oil and it's thousands of uses.

ADD and ADHD is just the beginning for me.

It goes so much deeper than that, and because it's in the news, it sells. Now people are starting to pay attention.

I guess it seems easy for the standard population to trust CBD if cancer patients are getting relief and results, especially because cancer is such a sensitive topic and somehow affects us all at some time in our lives in painful, painful ways.

Understandably, we as a population do not see the effects of ADHD as profound, but as I sat and catalogued the effects on Keagan's life, our lives, and others . . . I really had to take a bit of inventory.

So often individuals with ADHD turn to substances, alcohol, violence, painkillers, Ritalin, other mind-altering drugs . . . just to "cope".

Often, I have seen, heard and witnessed so many people discount the effects ADD or ADHD has on the individual. (And the family members.)

What they're not thought to be dying from is ADD or ADHD, or so people think. While numerous scientific studies have been done, it is still largely discounted that there is a significant increase in suicide rates among those diagnosed with ADHD.*

Further, what some don't take into consideration is all of the other conditions that someone experiences with ADD or ADHD and the domino effect that happens with it.

CHAPTER 6: WHAT IS IN STORE FOR CBD?

I truly believe CBD products will unfold in a very similar fashion that started around 2010 with the organic food industry.

Year over the year that industry doubled as more information and more education was made public or put into the mainstream media.

People started to realize that all of the pesticides and chemicals that are being put on their fruits and vegetables as well as consumed by the animals who would produce their meat supply.

As people began to realize how detrimental that was to them, the organic food industry took off, veganism took off, and people started speaking with their wallets.

Now people are starting to realize that big pharma and all of the chemicals that we're putting into our bodies for the symptoms that we're having isn't actually addressing the cause.

It is sick care, not healthcare.

And now more and more people are realizing that the CBD molecule in the plant is something that our body naturally needs and we're becoming more humble about accepting the fact that it is a natural substance and it is a natural plant.

Just because it's been labeled differently in the past doesn't mean it's any different from zucchini or a piece of broccoli.

What it does mean is that we do not need to take so many chemicals and so many versions of medicine that, again, just treat the symptoms and not the actual cause.

When given the right conditions, the entire body heals. I truly believe the body is capable of extraordinary things when given the ability to fight.

CHAPTER 7: ACCEPTING MY FAILURE & COMMITTING

I realized that I really started to open up my eyes to CBD and what it really was when I realized my ignorance, and my failures.

When I was learning more about CBD and what it was and how uneducated I was, that's when I realized, all of the failures, all my faults.

There were a million of them while I was raising my son. There were so many things I did wrong. There were so many things that I could have done better, and of course, there were some out of my control.

Of all I have been through in this life, this I feel is one of my biggest failures. Why?

I was so set in my ways. I was so closed off. I was so convinced.

I failed in a big way. And as a result, he suffered.

The more and more I became educated on the CBD products, the differences and the strains, and everything surrounding CBD, I knew there was so much more to learn.

I'm still learning, but I know I must bring this out to other people. I know so many people, including some family members, who struggle terribly with ADHD.

It's sad to watch people, mostly children, get treated differently. They get talked to differently, put into different programs, they're placed in different seating in the classroom, held back, given different work, etc...

I know there are parents that get phone calls from teachers and caregivers asking, "Did they miss their pill today?"

This breaks my heart. For the child and the parent.

If there's anything that I can do to help somebody receive more education or bring awareness to something that's natural, I will do everything I can.

My hope is to help them young, not be on drugs, not be medicated, not feel zombie-like, and not have to be different than everybody else.

I will do whatever I can to educate as many people as I can about not making the same mistakes I did.

CHAPTER 8: YOU'RE NOT ALONE IN YOUR SEARCH

I want people to be informed. I want people to know that there's many of us out there.

There are many of us out there that were misinformed, that were uneducated and were ignorant of what alternative methods could do for us and what they were.

So most importantly this is the impact that I want to make, education.

I don't think that others realize the effect and benefits that CBD can do and I also want others to know the side effects of the meds that they are on, as well as the benefit of using CBD as opposed to Ritalin or the like. The difference in side effects alone is immense. The side effects that are present with prescription drugs are tremendous.

People are given prescription drugs to help benefit many things that come with ADD/ADHD, such as imbalances, anxiety, depression, even more so than just coping with the condition alone.

The prescription drugs and having somebody feel the effects of years and years of prescription drugs in your system can be irreversible.

It's been associated with all sorts of other side effects that can happen from being on long term drugs, not to mention addiction.

You have peace of mind when you choose a natural product and knowing that CBD is not addictive, that there are no long-term side effects, and that you can't overdose is an easy decision to at least look into it.

Yes, one can be sensitive to CBD and it may not agree with them but that's no different then people being sensitive to eggs. It's the same type of thing; those long term side effects just aren't there with CBD.

Since my son never took medicine, the struggles were present every day, and because I chose not to put my son on Ritalin, his grades were lower, he failed classes, and he always had to be sent home with extra homework.

He struggled with classroom settings in general, being disruptive, issues with friends; following simple tasks . . . it was a constant for his entire adolescence.

I have also watched family members struggle while on and off Ritalin. It's heartbreaking.

CHAPTER 9: IF I HAD TO START ALL OVER AGAIN WITH EDUCATION SURROUNDING CBD (HERE'S WHAT I'D DO)

It's so difficult to see what position that put our children in, but - I get that it is REALLY EASY to do it. It is so easy to "follow the norm", but, what we have to pause for a moment and remember is . . . our children know.

They know that people are talking about them.

They know they are different.

I remember the conversation changing with my son as I became more educated.

I remember him telling me that he was taking oils and different remedies with other benefits to calm himself down to sleep, just to turn his brain off and sleep through the night.

He told me how he felt more at ease with himself, and so many other little private details that all related to a general sense of calm, a growing sense of being "okay" and that he finally felt like he was progressing.

I know that what Keagan went through destroyed his confidence, and the road ahead is still long.

It crushed him and brought out so many insecurities that I don't know if he'll ever fully recover from, but if he "feels better", if he feels like he is progressing, I am good with that.

If only this was 20 years ago. I'd turn back the clock and extract this damn oil myself.

CHAPTER 10: FOR THOSE CURIOUS ABOUT ALTERNATE METHODS FOR ADD/ADHD

I want to say, that It's not necessarily that people need to switch over to this new way of thinking, but more so that taking the time to look at CBD products differently is worth the time and energy investment.

There's nothing worse than seeing somebody that you love, in a state that literally alters them to the point where they're not themselves anymore.

When you notice that your child's energy, excitement and overall sense of well being is diminished, it is devastating.

They're resilient and they're genuinely happy. They haven't been tainted by other crap in the world when they're young and when you watch that diminish when you put your kid on a drug, and you watch them change, and change the person that they are, to me, that's worse.

If it's not necessary, it's heartbreaking, and I know for a fact, just the experiences with my son and my ex-husband, that they liked who they were.

I repeat they were. Not that they aren't incredible people, but circumstances in life can and do change you.

They really liked who they were and they're good people, but society kept telling them that they needed to be different.

So the fact that somebody could literally be taking a natural product and not have to change the human being that they are is incredible and worth researching.

CBD can regulate someone's mood and has a calming effect, it allows someone to think a little clearer and not get side tracked so easily.

This could help someone keep a job, or focus on reading a favorite book, or just simply completing a task.

I saw the struggles with all of the above daily, over and over again.

I'm not saying that there aren't millions of individuals out there that carry on a completely "normal" way of life while having ADD/ADHD and not being on medication, I'm just saying that there are alternatives worth looking into for those who need it.

You can't solely blame a condition on all of the mishaps, roadblocks, and failures that may happen in your life and I'm not naive, but there are things that I would have done differently.

There are opportunities that I missed and a better relationship that I would have had with both my ex-husband and my son.

Things were not handled properly when Keagan was young, and all of those social anxieties and everything else that came with it just carried forward in life because of it.

It's like being bullied by yourself your entire life, or a form of abuse. It's the same thing. People treat you differently if you're different.

You treat yourself differently if you feel you are different.

There are so many different side effects to prescription medicine... so really what are our choices?

Live with it or die from the prescriptions?

There are children still fighting and the struggles that they are going through is so hard to see and hear about, but in my heart, I truly think the day is coming where we will look at CBD no different than the way we look at constituents from any other plant.

I can't believe the change that I see in my son. It's like night and day. He's more relaxed, has more patience and is able to cope better with certain highs and lows.

It will never be what it could have been with Keagan, and he will never fully recover from the situations that he experienced, but he's able to manage it so much better now.

His relationships are stronger and he's able to focus on more of what he loves. He still games, a lot, as do 99% of those that I know with ADD and ADHD.

Something that I didn't discuss earlier on in this book that I think is very important to mention was the struggles that I had with both him and his father about gaming. I know that it seems so trivial but I never allowed it at our house because his Dad had all of the gaming equipment at his, and I wanted Keagan to go outside and play, to socialize and be active.

What I didn't see and believe, when he repeatedly told me these things, was that he felt at his best when he was gaming.

That's where he felt most comfortable and safe.

Their brains and their hands work so well together and they can synchronize their hands on those game controllers to the speed of that game.

They're in their element and they're in a safe place. I never understood that.

That was his outlet and favorite place to be, in the creative world of machines and animation.

Nobody judged him there, he was excellent at what he did and still does, and like-minded people surrounded him.

Another one of the biggest regrets was holding that from him when he was with me.

I simply share this to remind you, it is okay to change your mind. It is okay to have an opinion different than society.

CHAPTER 11: OUR BREAKTHROUGH

My son and I would talk about how he felt.

Finally, we could actually have conversations, and he didn't get so upset anymore. He didn't get as angry so quickly.

I noticed that he had more patience and that he was calmer and not always so quick to jump to a fight.

It was always an inner-struggle with him and I remember as I became more educated I reached out to my son and I said, "I need to understand more."

I remember him saying, "I never thought I'd see the day that my mom would phone me and ask me to talk to her about CBD and what it was that I was taking."

I never thought that I'd see the day that I went to my son for this reason. The simple fact that I went to my son for his advice and his experience on this taught me how well educated he was about it and how ignorant I was in judging so much about it and him.

My son was not somebody who just picked up a bottle of CBD oil and said, "Yeah, whatever, I'll give it a try and see what happens next."

My son dissected it. He researched it. He got to know exactly what it was and how it was made and where it was derived from.

He also researched what was best going to suit him and his struggles, even to the level of understanding the various types of plants.

When I was sitting there listening to my son talks about it, I felt like I was sitting there talking to somebody with a degree.

He really did his research. He really took it seriously and paid attention to it. He respects people's opinions and their differences surrounding it.

He knew that it was going to be a struggle. He knew that he was going to have a little bit of a fight, a bit of a controversy. He knew that he needed to be educated so he could back himself up.

Now, he was able to come back at somebody with an educated answer, and he takes that very seriously.

Seeing this transformation and newfound confidence . . . to a mom, priceless.

CHAPTER 12: SOURCES FOR THOSE CURIOUS ABOUT ALTERNATE METHODS FOR ADD/ADHD UPDATES AND NEWS

I really do see this becoming globally accepted.

I find that the more and more we start seeing common use of CBD.

As usual, it's not until we see the celebrities doing it, the doctors and the sports teams talking about it that we finally take the time to do our own research.

But, the more of a social spotlight that is put onto these natural products, and other natural remedies and methods, the more we as consumers are going to start speaking with our dollars.

The debates, the controversy, the quick to assume the conclusion . . . won't stop anytime soon. For over a century our society has looked at anything regarding the hemp plant as a risk.

If you take some time to research the history of tobacco, cotton, and hemp . . . you will quickly see that the reason the hemp plant was "discounted" was because of money. The hemp plant is easier to produce, grows faster and solves more problems than tobacco, (of course), and cotton.

But the true fact of that matter is this . . . tobacco and cotton cannot be easily grown by the common person. Whereas, a hemp plant can be, so what does that mean? That means that the "powers that be" couldn't monopolize profits.

Suddenly, hemp crops were replaced with cotton and tobacco crops. Paper and clothes were no longer made of hemp, they were now made of cotton.

I encourage any of my readers to check out some of the histories regarding how and why marijuana became illegal in Canada and the USA. It's both fascinating and mind-blowing at parts.

But, until we get educated as a society and rise above the corporations...

It's controversial.

Again, mark my words, it's going to be talked about even that much more.

We're going to be more educated ... we will keep using our dollars to have a voice, and I don't see this slowing down any time soon.

In fact, they're just going to keep coming out with more and more and more things that this is beneficial for, not only gaining focus and helping with anxieties.

CHAPTER 13: WHAT'S ON THE HORIZON FOR EDUCATION SURROUNDING CBD

One of the safest and more common ways to ingest or take CBD is orally, both in the oils and the drops and of course so many others say. There are edibles, cookies, vaping, and a long list of others ... I find that the oils, more so than not, are administered to children, at every age.

So from elderly to children, that is the most common, and in all different flavors. It's nice to see so many companies that are starting to do all sorts of amazing things with CBD oil now.

There are oils for pets, there are topical creams, face creams, pain creams, dog treats, mints, gummies, shampoos, tanning lotions and so much more.

Since it has the possibility to treat so many different things, people are finding clever and creative ways to have CBD in and around them.

One of the most common uses is also pain management. I have a friend who was hit head-on by a distracted driver and the amount of pain she deals with is extraordinary. She was able to have back surgery, but still deals with significant pain.

She uses the pain cream for her back instead of taking pain medication and that, to me, is a huge win.

I'm from Canada, and recently CBD has been in the news a lot. At the time of writing this book, we are only a few months post-Canada beginning to pass laws legalizing the use in some cases. Now the dispensaries are able to sell it to more people, not just the terminally ill.

There is still a lot of regulation as to where it's from, where it's grown, the types, and it's still causing a lot of controversies because crossing borders is an issue. It's still considered illegal in a lot of places, but it's getting better and the laws or changing.

We're still trying to iron all of that out, and there are a lot of gray areas, but the pages of laws that are available to read are endless.

I encourage you to read the documentation about the different types available, and THC, the different levels and what it's all used for, it really is interesting.

It's very important to know your facts when you're talking about the THC levels. Across the 50 states in the United States, it's legal, but in Canada, you have to be very specific about having particular reasons for the use.

So, stay tuned, this is still an ever-changing topic, with more and more insight being shared about it by the day.

CHAPTER 14: FINAL THOUGHTS & NEXT STEPS

After my hours and hours of research, after personally using CBD oils and creams myself, after seeing so many friends having success with ailments that negatively impacted themselves and their children, I decided I wanted to be a full-time supporter of more people learning of the CBD oil benefits.

I am not a homeopath, I am not a big-pharma lover, I am simply a logical person who seeks to understand and be resourceful and because of that, I will always support techniques and products that move us all forward, help us live a comfortable life, and most importantly achieve our goals.

At the time of sharing this chapter of my story with you, there are a number of ways for folks to enter the CBD world so if you are interested in using the products, becoming a distributor, or simply have questions - please do not hesitate to reach out to me at any time.

I can also be found at www.motivatedspaces.com

Stay Motivated, Stay Inspired, and Stay You!

Thank you for sticking with me until the end!!

Joelle Sloboda Mickelson

References:

Suicide and ADHD https://www.ncbi.nlm.nih.gov/pmc/articles/PMC5371172/